STOP SMOKING FAST:
15 WAYS THAT ACTUALLY WORK.
BONUS: 45 MORE HELPING MINI-MEHTODS

by Gary Pickler

I0416085

Stop Smoking Fast: 15 Ways That Actually Work

by Gary Pickler

Copyright © 2016, Gary Pickler

ISBN13: 978-1-329-84006-5

This book is not intended as medical advice. It's intent is solely informational and educational. Please, consult a health professional if you have questions about your health. The author and publisher are not liable for any damages or negative consequences from any treatment, action, application, or preparation, to any person reading or following the information in this book.

First Edition   : March 2016

Cover design   : Gary Pickler

Editing, proof reading, page design, book design

                         : Bruno Curfs

Publisher   : Gary Pickler, through Lulu

Table of Contents

Introduction

Many people seeing the title of my book may be shocked, at first. *Fifteen* different powerful ways! And, they *actually work*! Most other books claiming to stop smoking have only one way. And, often that "measly one way" either doesn't *really* work, or has a "catch".

Well, your smoking days are over, once you've bought this book and applied one of the fifteen methods. All the methods work, so it's your choice!

Actually, multiple methods of stopping smoking may *really* be necessary. Over and over, I hear of someone stopping smoking *only temporarily,* to then start again in several weeks, months, or years. Once they start smoking again, they may have lost confidence in the "stopping method" they used before.

The second time, they need a brand new method! With all the novelty and hope that a new method will bring! So, this is where *fifteen* different actually working methods come in handy. Whichever method you select, to stop smoking the first time, you'll have plenty of methods left, to stop a second or third time, etc., if necessary.

Hopefully, of course, the method you select the first time will permanently stop your smoking! But just in case some *accident* or *stressful life period* gets you started again, rest assured that you'll be able to pick a second method, to stop your smoking *again!*

Method #1, the "Silica System" (the method I start out with) is the *best*, I believe. It only requires that you eat ¾ cup of organic "quick oats" for breakfast, with raisins or dates. Then a sandwich of organic sprouted bread and cucumber slices (with their skin). The sandwich can be cheese, peanut butter, bologna, or whatever you like. Then one organic potato (with its skin) for dinner with whatever else you usually eat for dinner). That's it, essentially. All these foods are rich in the trace mineral *silica*, which has definitely proven to stop all craving for cigarettes.

My book explains Method #1 (the Silica System) at length, because most people need a *thorough explanation* before they'll consider changing their diet, to regularly include oats, sprouted bread, cucumbers (with skin) and potatoes (with skin). In addition, I found that turmeric powder is so important that I will periodically remind you to add it to your diet.

The other Methods #2 to #15 require *far* less explanation, because they are all fairly straight-forward.

At any rate, all fifteen methods work, so it's up to you to choose the method that appeals to you *most*, to successfully stop your smoking.

It is my wish that you quickly stop your smoking, and begin immediately to lead a much healthier and happier life!

Special Note

My book's purpose is to *stop your smoking, fast*, so that you'll be healthier and happier. This *brief* book, of useful instruction, will do exactly that, *in fifteen different ways*!

Two hundred more pages, of theory, philosophy, and rambling, are totally unnecessary. I've gotten right to the point, to avoid wasting your precious time!

Important Explanation Of The Silica System's Origin

This book is dedicated to Anthony Shkreli, the discoverer of the "Silica System": a system to stop smoking with silica rich foods. Every so often, a brilliant and creative man comes forward with an innovative solution to a worldwide problem. Anthony Shkreli is this great man! He has paved the way for millions of smokers to stop craving tobacco, and stop smoking, with his Silica System.

Anthony Shkreli has written two books on this Silica System. His first book is *You Are Not Addicted to Cigarette Smoking, You Are Starving* (for the silica mineral). His second book is *The Natural Cure For Cigarette Smoking* (which is silica). Anyone curious about the whole psychological and philosophical explanation, should buy and read these two interesting and *very detailed* books!

My book, based on Anthony Shkreli's Silica System gets right to the point about how to stop smoking fast, and thus omits 95% of Shkreli's complicated intellectualizations. It also features *fourteen* additional methods!

Obviously, if it weren't for Anthony Shkreli's two extremely explanatory books (of 208 pages and 56 pages, respectively), my brief book here, which is only a get-right-to-the-point summary, could never have existed! I am very grateful for Anthony Shkreli's discovery of the Silica System to stop smoking, which has enabled this brief fix-it-fast book to get out to the world, and help millions of smokers to stop smoking!

And, this is not all, for any great genius usually *continues* with their innovative, world-transforming ideas! If you are impressed with Anthony Shkreli's invention of a *fast* stop-smoking method, try reading his incredible third book *Seven Pillars Volume One*, in which he clearly shows you how to improve your life in many more ways, despite the limitations of what society teaches us.

Stop Smoking Fast!
How Eating Silica-Rich Foods
Stops Your Craving To Smoke!

Chapter 1 - The Silica System

Introduction

An incredibly amazing discovery has occurred, namely the "Silica System", that by eating foods rich in the mineral silica, all craving for smoking gradually disappears. This system truly, genuinely works, so that a cure for smoking has finally been found!

The mineral silica used to be plentifully supplied in our diet, a hundred and fifty years ago, before modern grain-milling industry began removing the fibrous bran part of the grain. What was left failed to adequately supply our silica mineral needs. As a result, most of us today are severely deficient in the mineral silica.

Silica is needed, and is even necessary, for the brain and body to function at top capacity. Silica is very important for thinking and memory, and low silica in the diet can make Alzheimer's disease three times as likely. Emphatically stated, silica really improves the mind and all mental functions.

The tobacco plant absorbs enormous amounts of silica from the soil. Thus, the tobacco plant is called, by botanists, a *silica accumulator.*

The actual reason why people smoke tobacco, is because of their *silica deficiency*! Tobacco supplies their silica nutritional requirement, but in a very harmful way, due to all the other unhealthy chemicals in tobacco products.

By eating foods rich in silica and/or by taking the very, very best silica supplements (such as turmeric powder capsules), you'll satisfy your silica nutritional need, and will then find that your desire for tobacco completely falls off! Since you'll be getting your needed silica from food or silica supplements, it won't be necessary to get your silica from tobacco products any more, and the tobacco craving will decrease over days, and be completely gone in a week or two. What a miracle this is!

The foods with the highest silica content are listed in Kaufmann's *Silica the Forgotten Nutrient*, numerically rated (on page 83). They are (with silica contents per 100 g [= 3.53 oz] servings): oats (595 mg), millet (500 mg), barley (233 mg), potatoes (200 mg), and whole wheat grains (158 mg). Also very high in silica are: cucumber (with its skin), bell peppers, rice, and especially turmeric powder. Kaufmann recommends 500-1000 mg of silica per day. It is highly recommended that you buy all these products in their *organic* form, in a *health food* store! By eating quite a bit of these 9 silica-rich foods, you should easily get the daily amount of silica needed to stop your tobacco cravings.

Silica System's Three Variations To Follow

Here follows a list of three variations of the Silica System.

1. A silica-rich food diet, using the 9 silica-rich foods listed above.

2. Taking four silica-rich herbs: oat straw, licorice root, echinacea, and sarsaparilla root.

Perhaps you can simmer them in a tea? This variation might not provide enough silica by itself, but can be used along with silica-rich foods, especially if you like tea a lot!

3. Silica supplements.

The taking of silica supplements is mentioned in Anthony Shkreli's book *The Natural Cure For Cigarette Smoking* on pages 46-48, 51-52.

When I first read this, it seemed that many types of silica supplements were available and that they all "worked". But what I found from *experimentation* was very disappointing! Silica supplements of "just the silica mineral" *did not* work, because *inorganic* silica, in an *unchelated* form, just forms a coating on the inside of your digestive tract and blood vessels, and will *not* be absorbed to have any real effect! I experienced this "inner coating" sensation, and it was unpleasant.

However, when I tried an *organic* form of silica (organic vegetal silica), that was *chelated*, as it was extracted from the *spring horsetail* plant (*equisetum arvense*), it apparently had some toxic residue of the plant! I had an allergic reaction to it causing extreme fatigue, nausea, and lasting kidney pain! Neither did it work for two of my friends; both also had an allergic reaction. My friends and I are highly sensitive people. Perhaps "organic vegetal silica" supplements can be taken by people who don't respond allergically to it.

Silica *gel* capsules are also referred to as "colloidal silica", which have *billions* of tiny particles that go through cell walls. Because of the above, I speculate that silica gel, which is inorganic and unchelated, cannot be absorbed.

Anyway, it *seems* that we must get our silica from *foods*, and not from supplements! The exception is to take turmeric powder or turmeric powder capsules with meals, which work really well! (See the section Turmeric-Powder-Power in Chapter 2).

Practical Guidelines

It may get tiresome, over time, to keep ingesting silica every day, but this is the "price you'll need to pay", to continue having *no craving to smoke*! Also, remember that the silica mineral is really good for your health, anyway!

As you use the Silica System to supplement your body (and brain), with silica, you'll find that your craving for smoking and tobacco products will gradually taper off. Interestingly, your *sugar* craving may be reduced too, because many silica-starved people yearn for sugar (because sugar contains a very small percentage of silica, from its refining process). How many overweight sugar-addicts are really (unknowingly) trying to satisfy their *silica* deprivation? Wouldn't it be great if you lost a lot of weight (from reduced sugar craving) after regularly ingesting silica, daily? Also, you'll probably find that silica sharpens your mind and memory significantly!

Some people trying this Silica System, by eating lots of silica-rich foods, have stopped all desire for smoking in just days! Incredible, right? Others took a week or two, before their craving for smoking stopped. It's not really necessary, with the Silica System, to "try" to stop smoking. No, just regularly ingest plenty of silica daily, and the urge to smoke will just slowly subside on its own!

Once you have no more craving to smoke, you've done it. You've won! No more smoking! But, of course, you'll still have to continue your daily silica ingestion, or a returned deficiency of silica will start up your craving to smoke again.

We can all be incredibly grateful to the brilliant discoveries and inventor of the Silica System, Anthony Shkreli! Highly recommended are Anthony Shkreli's two books on all this, *The Natural Cure For Cigarette Smoking* (silica), and *You are Not Addicted, You Are Starving* (for silica). These two books contain many, many more details of it all than my brief summary here. Buy them!

Conclusion

I realize that many people may be very skeptical about this brief summary, but, really, it works! Experiment with it! You've got very little to lose, by buying some silica rich foods (all cheap), at an organic health food store, eating them, filling yourself up with silica and experiencing the very healthful results. And when it all works for you, then you'll have kicked smoking forever.

Besides stopping your craving for cigarettes, silica may greatly reduce your sugar craving and your waistline, while silica keeps your mind and memory strong!

Chapter 2 - Silica And Nutrition

100 Nutrients Needed

Silica by itself will stop your craving to smoke, but for building excellent health, approximately *100* nutrients are needed by everyone's body! If anyone is deficient in any one of these 100 nutrients, a reduction in their healthiness will eventually start to be felt! So obviously, try to eat the healthiest diet possible, and consider taking vitamin and mineral supplements.

Stress Requires Even More Nutrients

When people go through stress in their lives, they usually need even *more* nutrients than usual! It's as if stress is like a modern era "plague", that requires tip-top nutrition, to handle all this stress. Eating lots of silica-rich foods enables you to handle modern day stress much easier! It's almost as if the mineral silica is an anti stress nutrient.

Nourishing Your Cells Is Most Important

Most people eat food today for its taste, and to fill up their stomach. But the most important reason for eating, is to *nourish* your cells! The best way to do this, is to regard your cells as "babies", that need "baby-food". Lots of chewing, of the most nutritious foods (plus silica) enables the best digestion and the best nourishment of your "baby" cells, to give you energy!

Your Brain's Great Silica Need

The scientist Edith Carlyle, in her book *Silicon Biochemistry*, notes that many areas of the brain need a high degree of silica concentration, to function at peak brain efficiency.

Turmeric-Powder-Power!

The turmeric plant is a silica accumulator (from the soil). Thus, eating turmeric powder—organic is best, sold in many health food stores—gives you a great deal of silica, besides the very beneficial curcumin in it.

This is such an important supplement that I strongly advise including turmeric powder with each meal, so that its silica is spread out over the day. Two level tea spoons of turmeric powder—sprinkled on food, or mixed with a sauce— should be enough. If you don't like the taste of turmeric powder, then take 3 times a day 5 large size turmeric capsules with food. Alternatively, stir 2 level tea spoons of turmeric powder in a glass of juice, tea, or cold water, and quickly swallow it down, then rinse out your mouth.

Brain Very Affected By Silica-Deficiency

Deficiency of silica adversely affects the brain, by making it very hard for neurotransmitters to cross neuronal synapses in the brain!

Bran And Hull: Very, Very Silica-Rich!

Bran and hull (as in oat bran, wheat bran, corn bran, and rice bran) are very, very rich in silica. When you eat sprouted whole grain bread, try adding these brans too, to enrich your silica-meal even more! After all, we all became deficient in silica, by having these silica-rich brans *subtracted* from our grains. So, try doing the *opposite*, by adding back even more bran, and raw (or toasted) wheat germ! By this, you create "silica-enriched" whole grain sprouted bread! I eat the brans and wheat germ raw, with the whole wheat bread.

Biggest Enemies Of Silica Absorption

These are the worst "stoppers" of absorbing silica:

1. *Aluminum*. Aluminum is toxic, and "pushes out" silica, so that the silica isn't absorbed! Try to reduce your intake of aluminum as much as possible. Don't use aluminum cooking pots, or drink soda pop from aluminum cans. Live in an area where airplanes aren't spraying "chem trails" of aluminum particles way up in the sky, which will eventually fall down (from high overhead) into your lungs and body, wrecking your silica absorption and health.[1]

2. *Stress*. Reduce stress in your life as much as possible. Or even double your silica intake, to help you deal with all this stress.

3. *Sugar*, white bread, and refined grains, which practically do the *opposite* of silica, and cause many immediate and long term bad health problems. Cut down on them!

4. *Antibiotics*. These kill of your intestinal probiotics, so that vitamin B3 absorption is interfered with. Since vitamin B3 is a great *helper* of silica absorption, the

---

1 Cf. http://www.ncbi.nlm.nih.gov/pubmed/19064650.

wrecking of vitamin B3 absorption by antibiotics will greatly hurt silica absorption.

A "Silica Reserve" Is The Goal

Once you start silica ingestion, from silica-rich foods, your health and energy should gradually get better and better, until you've built up a "silica reserve", that you should try to maintain by continued daily silica ingestion. This "saturation with silica" is what will cause you to lose your craving for cigarettes, and be much healthier, mentally and physically.

Vitamin B3, In A Vitamin B Complex, Is A Big "Helper" To Silica

Vitamin B3 tremendously helps the assimilation of silica, and thus *could* be taken too, to speed up this whole process! But because the B-vitamins all work together as a "team", *all eleven* B-vitamins are necessary (in this remedy, to stop smoking). Vitamins B1 (thiamin), B2 (riboflavin), B3 (niacin or niacinamide), choline (formerly B4), B5 (pantothenic acid), B6 (pyridoxine, pyridoxal, pyridoxamine), B7 (biotin), B8 (inositol), B9 (folic acid), B10 (PABA or para-amino-benzoic acid), B12 (cobalamins, such as cyanocobalamin) are all necessary, to be present, in the vitamin B complex. If even *one* of these eleven B-vitamins are missing, then find *another* brand of vitamin B complex, with *all these eleven* B-vitamins in it. This is very, very important! If you neglect this, and if even *one* B-vitamin is missing, then you'll gradually become deficient in the missing B-vitamin, and the whole remedy will be wrecked! Deficiency in the missing B-vitamin usually causes a type of "unexplained fatigue" I've found from experience.

Also, the vitamin B3 in the B complex capsule needs to be vitamin B3 in the form of niacinamide and *not* niacin. This is because vitamin B3 as niacin causes an itchy, red, unpleasant flush in the face and all over the body. To prevent this extreme flushing irritation, vitamin B3 as niacinamide (and *not* niacin) should be taken. A good brand of multiple B vitamins, for only $7.99, is *Solaray B-Complex 50* in a 50 capsule bottle. It can be ordered at http://www.solaray.com/ or by phoning 1 (800) 683-9640. Solaray B-complex 50 is highly recommended, since it has all the above requirements and is inexpensive!

Remember, though, that it's really silica that stops the smoking. Vitamin B3 (in a vitamin B complex) is just a "helper". But still, I highly recommend taking a vitamin B complex with the silica-rich foods!

Silica Is A Needed, Required Nutrient For Health

Even if you were not a smoker (and using silica to stop smoking), you would still need plenty of silica for your health! Silica is such a needed nutrient, and all people living in our modern civilization are so *silica-deficient*, that it can confidently be said that silica ingestion can solve many of your problems resulting from this silica-deficiency! Thus, silica is the key to not only stopping smoking, but to building the "super-health" that we all desire!

Gary Pickler

Chapter 3 - Numerous Silica Health Benefits

Silica is not "just another trace mineral", to continue to ignore. Instead, silica *very powerfully* promotes overall good health! Silica helps you to stay younger longer, and stops "early aging". Wounds heal much faster with silica. Bone and connective tissue, especially collagen, build more rapidly with silica. Silica helps to stop Alzheimer's disease, and prevents cardiovascular disease! Silica-rich foods and silica supplements revitalize your skin, hair, and nails, to make you look much younger, too!

Silica stimulates growth in bone fractures. Silica helps create healthy arteries. Silica helps the body to manage and balance water. Silica attracts many much-needed minerals. Silica balances pH. Silica greatly benefits the brain and cognitive behavior. Silica greatly reduces stress.

Obviously, all these incredible benefits mean that it *really makes sense* to eat plenty of silica-rich foods, to greatly enhance your overall good health (besides stopping your craving to smoke)!

These three books (available on the internet) go into *much greater detail* on the utterly amazing benefits of silica. They are (1) *Silica The Forgotten Nutrient* (106 pp.) and (2) *Silica, The Amazing Gel* (159 pp.), both by Klaus Kaufmann, and (3) *Silica* (46 pp.) by Edward A. Lemmo, Ph.D.

Get and read these three books, if you're still not convinced of the extraordinary health benefits of silica!

Gary Pickler

Chapter 4 - Silica Plans

Plan A

(From Anthony Shkreli's book *The Natural Cure for Cigarette Smoking*, pp. 35, 40-41.)

During the course of your day, eat *four* cucumbers (organic is best), including their skin. (The silica is in the skin.) Eat four cucumbers in various ways throughout your day, perhaps in a salad with dressing, or in a sandwich, or put in a blender (with other greens). Use your imagination, and invent your own "Cucumber Ultra Delight" recipe! To avoid getting "bored" with all these cucumbers, try combining them with as many other tasty foods as you can! Remember, never peel their silica-rich skin, unless you plan to eat only the skin. Four cucumbers a day will do it, to *gradually* reduce your craving to smoke cigarettes to zero over the course of two weeks.

Plan B

(From Anthony Shkreli's book *The Natural Cure for Cigarette Smoking*, pp. 44-46.)

During the course of your day, eat *five* pieces (slices) of sprouted whole-grain bread, with butter. Toasting the bread is okay. Perhaps, eat two slices of buttered bread for breakfast. Then, for lunch or dinner, eat two more buttered slices. Finally, another buttered piece at bedtime, or late at night. The reason for the butter is that scientific studies have shown that butter or any other *saturated* fat, tremendously helps mineral absorption in people's bodies. (The same studies showed that *unsaturated* fats did not help at all.) Butter is best, but any other *saturated* fat will do, instead. Anyway, eat *some* kind of *saturated* fat, with the sprouted bread, to boost silica mineral absorption: cottage cheese, cheese, whole milk, yoghurt, coconut milk, organic nuts or organic nut butter. It's your choice.

If you don't want to eat a *saturated* fat with the sprouted bread, then you have to eat *twice* as much bread. Without the saturated fat, *ten* slices of sprouted bread per day are needed for the same result!

Incidentally, I've found that "Food For Life"-brand's "Genesis 1:29 Bread" and "Ezekiel 4:9 Bread" are *incredibly delicious* and nutritious! See the nutritional values of "Genesis 1:29 Bread" (Fig. 1) and "Ezekiel 4:9 Bread" (Fig. 2) on the next page.

These types of bread can be found in the "refrigerated bread section" of health food stores. And don't be put off by the "Genesis" and "Ezekiel"; obviously, eating an *amazingly tasty* bread, is not necessarily connected to religion.

Nutrition Facts

Serving Size 1 Slice (34g)
Servings Per Container About 20

Calories 80
Calories from Fat 15
Calories from Saturated Fat 0

* Percent Daily Values are based on a 2,000 calorie diet.

Amount/Serving	% Daily Value*	Amount/Serving	% Daily Value*
Total Fat 2g	3%	**Total Carb.** 14g	5%
Saturated Fat 0g	2%	Dietary fiber 3g	11%
Trans Fat 0g		Sugars 0g	
Cholesterol 0mg	0%	**Protein** 4g	8%
Sodium 65mg	3%	**Potassium** 100mg	

Vitamin A 0% • Vitamin C 0% • Calcium 0% • Iron 6%
Thiamine 10% • Magnesium 10% • Niacin 10% • Vitamin B6 4%
Riboflavin 2% • Phosphorus 10% • Zinc 4% • Folic Acid 4%

Fig. 1 - Nutritional value of "Genesis 1:29 Bread"

Nutrition Facts	Amount/Serving	% Daily Value*	Amount/Serving	% Daily Value*
Serving Size 1 Slice (34g) Servings Per Container About 20	**Total Fat** 0.5g	1%	**Total Carb.** 15g	5%
	Saturated Fat 0g	1%	Dietary fiber 3g	10%
	Trans Fat 0g		Sugars 0g	
Calories 80	**Cholesterol** 0mg	0%	**Protein** 4g	8%
Calories from Fat 5	**Sodium** 0mg	0%	**Potassium** 75mg	
Calories from Saturated Fat 0				

Vitamin A 0%	• Vitamin C 0%	• Calcium 0%	• Iron 4%
Thiamine 8%	• Magnesium 6%	• Niacin 6%	• Vitamin B6 4%
Riboflavin 2%	• Phosphurus 8%	• Zinc 4%	• Folic Acid 0%

* Percent Daily Values are based on a 2,000 calorie diet.

Fig. 2 - Nutritional value of "Ezekiel 4:9 Bread"

Plan C

Combine Plan A with Plan B! Eat four cucumbers and five slices of buttered, sprouted bread every day! One possibility here is four different types of sandwiches every day, each with (toasted?) buttered bread and cucumber slices. For the super-ambitious person, who wants to stop smoking *fast*!

Plan D

Add turmeric capsules to Plan A, Plan B or Plan C. See also the section Turmeric-Powder-Power in Chapter 2.

Gary Pickler

Chapter 5 - Final Thoughts

You have now finished reading about how the Silica System will stop your smoking. Also, I have told you just how to do it, with a few variations.

Now, the question is, are you going to do it? I really, really hope you do, and stop your smoking, and begin living a much healthier life!

But, people are very complicated psychologically, I've found, over many, many years. And often, at a point like this, people come up with all sorts of reasons and excuses *not* to do the thing next most indicated.

A "silver-tongued salesman" often walks in now, to "close the deal"! A stream of glib words, carefully chosen, to fill you up with extreme enthusiasm to try the Silica System (or some other kind of "sales abracadabra").

But the trouble is, I'm *not* any kind of salesman or promoter. Sorry! I *don't have* the "magic words" to transform you from a "reader" into a "Silica System Trier" (which will then result in your stopping smoking.)

So, I wonder if you'd do me a small favor. Could you bring onto the stage of your "inner psyche", *your own* Inner Salesman/Promoter? What would *your own* Salesman/ Promoter say to you right now? What "wise words of wisdom" seem to come into your mind now, encouraging you to give the Silica System an honest try?

Perhaps Inwardly You Hear

(1) "Boy, this silica thing is interesting. I wonder if it works? If it does, it would be great! But if it doesn't, I am *so tired* of trying these "stop-smoking things" that don't work! But this "silica thing" only involves eating four cucumbers (with their skin) every day. Or else, eating five slices of sprouted whole grain bread, with butter, every day. These two plans seem pretty simple! And cucumbers and sprouted bread are both good for me, anyway. Okay! Why don't I give this "cucumbers or bread-and-butter"-thing a try, for just *two weeks*, and see what happens?

Or perhaps inwardly you hear

(2) Something else!

Obviously, every single person reading this short book is *unique*, and I have *no* idea what's going on inside you, now. Also, not being any kind of salesman, I have no idea what to *say* to you anyway, about what's going on within you, now.

But please, could you just *try* this Silica System? From my heart, I'd really like you to stop smoking and begin to live a more wonderful life! And then tell your friends, who will listen to you, so that they'll try the Silica System too, and then they will tell *their* friends!

I care about you, and I want very much for the Silica System to stop your smoking, if you truly want this, too.

Anyway, if it just so happens that you *do* try the Silica System for two weeks, I would really like to hear about your results, *whatever they are*. Please, send me your results to my email: **garypickler1@gmail.com**. Thank you, thank you so much, for trying the Silica System, passing it on, and helping to heal more and more people from their smoking!

Gary Pickler

Chapter 6 - Fourteen Other Methods

Method #2 - Sicken Yourself With Cigs

This is a method where you literally make yourself *sick* with cigarettes and tobacco. You over-smoke and over-irritate yourself with tobacco and cigarettes until you utterly *hate them*!

This method is outlined in navy man Vince Stead's brief book *How I Stopped On My Own After Smoking A Pack A Day For 23 Years*. Vince Stead also has an e-book on this at a cheaper price.

This "Method #2" *actually works*, too, but requires that you've "got what it takes", to stick with this "self-tormenting-with-cigs" program, until you *hate* cigarettes enough to quit! Military dudes, and tough people with lots of willpower might prefer this method to the Silica System or else find a way to *combine* this "tough way" with eating silica-rich foods!

A more sophisticated version of this "Sicken Yourself With Cigs" method is also in Stewart Blackburn's book *The Skills of Pleasure-Crafting the Life You Want*, on pages 46-47. (This book is also available, more cheaply, as an e-book.)

Method #3 - Affirm Quitting Date Repeatedly, As One Smokes Heavily And Excessively

A friend of mine, Eliot, successfully quit in a similar way. For a whole year, from Jan. 1 to Dec. 31, he smoked heavily and even *excessively*. But, as he "puffed and puffed" on each cigarette, he affirmed, with certainty "I will be quitting on January 1st" (of the next year).

Thus, hundreds of times a day for 365 straight days, *with each cigarette as he smoked it,* he fervently declared, over and over, his *conviction* to quit at the beginning of the next year. Finally, when January 1st of the next year came, all his passionate affirming paid off, and he quit!

Method #4 - Very Gradual Reduction Of "The Patch"

Eliot's wife quit by slowly reducing "the patch", little by little, over seven weeks. Each day she would put on a smaller and smaller patch until there was no patch left, and she had quit. She distracted herself from cigarette cravings with (1) a glass of water, (2) a walk, (3) deep breathing, (4) sucking on straws or pencils (since smoking can be such an "oral" fixation).

Obviously, this method of gradually "reducing the patch", can be combined with eating silica-rich foods, too!

Also, this Method #4 can proceed even more slowly, to extend over several months, if necessary.

Method #5 - "Weaning"

(For those who want to stop tobacco, but keep smoking an "herbal blend".)

In Hilo, Hawai'i, a woman, Adah Glasser, operates a smoke shop called "Hilo Tobacco Company". Adah can be reached at 1 (808) 769-0324, Sunday–Thursday 12–5 (Hawai'i Time). Adah has a PayPal account for credit card transactions.

Adah sells an "herbal smoking blend" called "Awa of the Goddess". ½ ounce is $6.00 (plus $3.00 handling, and $6.00 shipping, if Adah has to mail it to you.)

During week 1, you smoke a mixture of 75% of your favorite tobacco and 25% "Awa of the Goddess". During week 2, you smoke a mixture of 50% tobacco and 50% "Awa". During week 3, you smoke a mixture of 25% tobacco and 75% "Awa". Then, during week 4, you smoke 100% "Awa" and you've quit your tobacco habit!

This Method #5 is called "Weaning", because, over four week, you've "weaned" yourself off tobacco. Of course, anyone trying this "Weaning" method can switch (to more and more "Awa") at a *slower* pace, or can even stop at 50% tobacco/50% "Awa", or stop at 25% tobacco/75% "Awa".

Method #6 - Top Notch, Competent Counseling

Adah Glasser is a very wise, compassionate, counselor for people who smoke tobacco and want to quit. Adah is very experienced in counseling hundreds of people. Ada charges $20 / ½ hour, or $40 / hour for over-the phone counseling at 1 (808) 769-0324 Sunday–Thursday 12–5 (Hawai'i Time). Adah has a PayPal account for credit card transactions.

After counselling hundreds of people on quitting cigarettes, Adah emphasizes:

(1) You need to be *really clear* about *why* you're quitting.

(2) If your act of quitting is not for *yourself*, it's not going to work! (In other words, quitting for your relationship

partner, or for your parents, or for your children, etc. seldom works.)

(3) If you quit for many months, then smoke just *one* cigarette, *don't* then "get into guilt", think "you've failed", and go back to smoking! No! You've quit for months, and one little cigarette is irrelevant (as long as you go back to having quit)!

(4) Combine this with Method #7, *lobelia*.

Anyway, Adah is available for "tobacco quitting counseling", if you're interested. Combining "Weaning" with her counselling is possible, too!

Method #5, the "Weaning" method, *actually works*, to gradually stop, or cut down, your tobacco. It is absolutely, definitely worth a try!

It's also possible to combine the Silica System with the "Weaning" method. When your silica nutrient needs are being met by *diet* (instead of by tobacco smoking), it's far easier to switch to smoking a delightful herbal blend, instead! Incidentally, Adah also mixes up a *whole variety* of really nice herbal blends, for smoking pleasure. Phone her, and ask about them!

Method #7 - Lobelia

Smoking *Lobelia* (or Indian Tobacco) fills in neuro-receptor sites and takes craving away. It is a much healthier herb to smoke than commercial cigarettes. (See Mini-Method #24.)

Method #8 - Herbal Blends

Experiment with smoking a whole variety of other really nice herbal blends to reduce your craving. (See Mini-Method #17.)

Method #9 - Herbal Tea Of Silica-Rich Herbs

Still another possibility is to get your silica nutrient from drinking a *tea* of oat straw, licorice root, echinacea, and sarsaparilla root (all silica-rich herbs). Add some turmeric powder to the tea. Then smoke your favorite herbal blend (without any tobacco in it), to satisfy your smoking pleasure! Also, some *lobelia* (Indian tobacco) can be smoked a bit too, which fills the neuro-receptor sites to take away tobacco craving. Thus you'll substitute for unhealthy tobacco: (1) a healthy herbal tea, (2) healthy turmeric powder, and (3) a healthy herbal blend to smoke (with perhaps *lobelia* thrown in there too). By doing it this way, you won't have to change your diet at all, and you'll be able to continue smoking (a non-tobacco delightful herbal blend).

Method #10 - Stop In 3 Days: Methods #1 through #9 combined

This is the "stop in three days" *super-fast formula*, for those who have little patience:

(1) Eat *five* slices of buttered whole-grain sprouted bread each day.
(2) Eat *four* organic cucumbers (with their skin on), each day.

(3) Brew four herbs, i.e., oat straw, licorice root, echinacea, and sarsaparilla root (all silica-rich herbs) into a tea, and drink several times a day.

(4) Smoke *lobelia* (Indian tobacco), instead of your usual cigarettes, so that the *lobelia* fills in the neuro-receptor sites and takes craving away (from regular tobacco, with all its unhealthy chemicals).

(5) Eat as much turmeric powder, with other food, as you can, without straining yourself too much. (Turmeric is very silica-rich.)

(6) Take one capsule, each day, of "Solaray B-Complex 50", as explained in Chapter 2. (Best taken with either the bread or cucumbers.) The vitamin B3 in this capsule originally was named *nicotinic acid*, when it was discovered in 1867 by the *chemical oxidation of nicotine*! This is all explained in great detail, in Anthony Shkreli's *You Are Not Addicted to Cigarette Smoking, You Are Starving*, on page 118-130. The bottom line is that "nicotinic acid" (*vitamin B3*) *acts the same way in the body as the* "nicotine" *from cigarettes*! So, essentially, you'll be getting the cigarette's silica from (1) to (5) listed above, and you'll be getting the cigarette's *nicotine* from "nicotinic acid" (vitamin B3) and *lobelia* (Indian tobacco).

These six actions, all powerfully put together like this, fervently done with the tough, militant will power displayed in Chapter 6's Method #2, should very effectively do the job—fast—in either one, two, or three days! At any rate, continue until there's no more craving for cigarettes. Then you can taper off the *lobelia* (Indian tobacco) gradually, until you're either not smoking *anything*, or else you've switched to smoking a delightful herbal blend, that you greatly enjoy! Perhaps you can "wean" yourself off the *lobelia* with gradual substitution of "Awa of the Goddess", as described in Chapter 7.

Adah's "herbal smoking blend", called "Awa of the Goddess", and her whole variety of other really nice herbal blends, and her wise, compassionate counseling at $20 / ½ hour, can really help you with your quitting process, here!

Method #11 - The Limit Of 7-A-Day System

My friend Karen was in her fifties, and had been smoking cigarettes for thirty years. She knew that dire health problems could begin, if she didn't quit, at her age.

Karen still enjoyed smoking a certain amount, however. So Karen decided on a plan to limit herself to *seven* cigarettes a day. But every day, after her seventh cigarette, Karen continued to smoke several more, and averaged about fifteen cigarettes a day (instead of seven). However, this still was better than the pack-of-20 Karen used to smoke, every day!

After Karen's seventh cigarette, she usually tried as hard as she could, with all her willpower, to stop for the day. So that, even though Karen smoked several more cigarettes than seven, she was still "exercising" her willpower "muscles", by trying to stop at seven!

Six months passed like this, and Karen became very disappointed in herself for "failing" every day, to stop at seven cigarettes only. At this point, Karen decided that her "Limit of

7-a-day System" just wasn't working. But she still knew that she needed to quit for health reasons.

Karen, at this point, decided to go "cold turkey". Not knowing of any other systems to stop cigarettes, Karen made a "capital D" *D*ecision to totally stop. And, she did! She was able, at this point, to completely stop smoking, and she had no nicotine withdrawal problems, and is still not smoking today, after all these years. So, Karen did it. She stopped!

Perhaps Karen's exercising of her willpower "muscles", every day for six months, developed these "muscles" enough so that Karen's will power (after six months of growing stronger) was finally strong enough to quit smoking altogether!

Method #12 - The Fear-Of-Death Method

Joe, the father of my best friend, had been a moderate smoker for 40 years. He was having severe heart pains, at the age of 66. When he went to see his doctor about it, his doctor did all the usual examinations and tests, then advised triple-bypass heart surgery. Joe was put in a hospital on a strict diet, and told not to smoke, for three weeks. This was because smoking would interfere with the upcoming operation.

Joe, at this point, had these three choices:

1. He could stop smoking, like the doctor ordered, for three weeks.

2. He could sneak outside the hospital, and smoke "on the sly", even though this could result in his *death*, from an unsuccessful operation.

3. He could leave the hospital, not have the operation, and risk death from an eventual heart attack.

But Joe had an important *reason* to stay alive! This was that he had just become a *grandfather*, and *loved* playing with his little granddaughter. It was *this*, that made Joe decide—while in the hospital, using all his will power—to quit smoking for three weeks.

Joe's operation was successful, and he went home afterward. And then he found that his three weeks of quitting smoking, as he waited in the hospital, had "done the job". Joe had no more desire to smoke, and now smoke-free, he could resume joyously playing with his little granddaughter!

The *essence* of this method is: become super-aware of possible death (from smoking), due to cancer, heart attack, or some other disease. Then, go to some "retreat space", and perhaps in isolation, stop smoking, over three weeks.

Try to do what Joe did:

1. Face the "smoker's death threat."

2. Decide exactly *why* you want to keep living, to give you the inspiration to stay alive!

3. *Decide* to quit, over the next three weeks.

4. Find a *place* to do this quitting, over three weeks, that will work for you.

5. *Quit*, by carrying out your plan!

6. Lavishly reward yourself, after quitting, by spending plenty of time doing exactly those things that motivated you to quite smoking, and stay alive.

That's it—the *"Fear-of-Death Method"* that worked for Joe! Alter this method, in any way you see fit, to specially tailor it to fit you and your circumstances.

Good luck!

Method #13 - The Hypnotic Ultra-Disgust Method

This method involves your going into a hypnotic trance, and having numerous "true negatives" (about cigarettes) suggested to you. The object is to fill you so full of *"ultra-disgust"* toward cigarettes, that you'll stop smoking!

With the hypnotic words of this method, possibility #1 is to record them into a recording device[2]. Then, later, when you're lying down, with eyes closed, and ready to be hypnotized, you can play all the recorded hypnotic words back, to yourself. Possibility #2 is to have *another person* (a friend) read—from this book—the hypnotic words to you when you're lying down with your eyes closed[3]. Either way is okay; it's up to you.

Before I write down the hypnotic words for you to use, it will greatly help for you to do a computer search for: "spittoon wild west saloon". Click on where it offers "spittoon *symbols*", then take a look at the pictures of actual, genuine *spittoons*, from the "wild west saloon" era. For, it will be *this spittoon* (in

---

2 It helps greatly to speak the words *slowly* and in a somewhat *monotone* voice.

3 Your friend should read the hypnotic words *slowly*!

your imagination, while hypnotized) that you will disgustingly place your face in! This repulsive placing of your face into the spittoon (full of cowboy tobacco juice spit, and raunchy cigarette butts) will be hypnotically associated with smoking. And, this awful experience is designed to fill you full of *utter disgust toward cigarettes* (to make you stop smoking)!

So now, go ahead and just read these words, designed to (later!) hypnotize you. *See* whether you (later) want to put yourself through this "ultra-disgusting" hypnotic experience, in order to stop your smoking! (If you don't, that's okay. Simply go on to one of the other methods in this book.)

HYPNOTIC WORDS THAT YOU'LL BE RECORDING, OR THAT YOUR FRIEND WILL READ TO YOU:

(START, remember to read slowly)

"Relax your entire body. Your entire body feels completely comfortable and relaxed. Relax your *feet*. Your feet feel completely comfortable and relaxed. Relax your *legs*. Your legs feel completely comfortable, and relaxed. Relax your *hips*. Your hips feel completely comfortable and relaxed. Relax your *stomach*. Your stomach feels completely comfortable, and relaxed. Relax your *chest*. Your chest feels completely comfortable, and relaxed. Relax your *arms*. Your arms feel completely comfortable, and relaxed. Relax your *hands*. Relax your *fingers*. Relax your *neck & throat*. Your neck & throat feel completely comfortable, and relaxed. Relax your *face* and your *head*. Your face, and your head, feel completely comfortable, and relaxed. Relax your *eyes*. Relax your *mouth*. Relax your entire body. Your entire body feels completely comfortable and relaxed. And, every breath that you take, makes you feel more comfortable and relaxed. Just lie there, and feel how good it feels, to feel so comfortable and relaxed. And every breath that you take, makes you feel more and more comfortable, and more and more relaxed.

(Now, record all these 172 "relax-relax-relax" words all over again, a second time, before proceeding *onwards*.)

"*Now*, I want you to fully open your mind and emotions, all the way, in listening to all the *truths* I will now tell you about cigarettes. I'm now going to tell you many, many *truths* about cigarettes that will flow straight into your mind and emotions *without any resistance*. Okay, here I go. Now, *absorb fully* all I'm going to say *directly* to you, about cigarettes, right now!"

(Pause 5 seconds.)

"Cigarettes are practically pure poison! They're full of hundreds of toxic chemicals that can wreck your health! Cigarettes can make you sick! They can destroy your energy and wreck your life! Cigarettes are like a demon that has gotten possession of you! When you smoke, you're like an enslaved drug addict, to nicotine! Smoking can kill you, and cause your death, if you continue! Continuing smoking could likely give you cancer, or a heart attack! Smoking has terrible health risks, and can systematically destroy your body! The smoking addiction can cause you sheer hell! When you smoke, you're suffocating yourself! The cost of a pack-a-day, over your whole life, is about a quarter of a million dollars! Society's brainwashing, that smoking is "cool", or "tough", is false! It's *non-smoking* that gives you health, happiness, and freedom from addiction! So, quit! Now that you see how terribly awful smoking is, from all these reasons, you'll feel so *disgusted* from smoking that you'll quit! Immediately! you'll completely stop your smoking, right now! You feel so *disgusted* toward cigarettes! Yes, you'll *stop*, and stop smoking, right *now*!

(Now, record the last two paragraphs, of 243 words total, all over again, a second time, before proceeding further.)

"Okay, now I want you to imagine that you're back in the "wild west days", around the year 1880. And, imagine that you're in a wild west saloon, full of cowboys. Let your imagination take you back through time, to around the year 1880, where you're standing inside an old wild west saloon, full of cowboys."

(Pause 5 seconds.)

"Okay, now look towards the bar, of the saloon, and in the middle of the bar, on the floor, see an old wild west *spittoon*. See this dirty, old, stinking spittoon, on the floor, in the middle of the bar."

(Pause 5 seconds.)

"Now, notice how all the cowboys are frequently "hawking" and *spitting* into the spittoon, and are often spitting out jets of chewing tobacco juice into the spittoon. See that the spittoon's outer surface is all covered with disgusting spit."

(Pause 5 seconds.)

"And notice also, that the spittoon is full of a few dozen raunchy cigarette butts, disgustingly floating in all the spit. See and picture this clearly."

(Pause 5 seconds.)

"Now, I want you to ignore all the cowboys, and walk up to the spittoon, so that you're standing right in front of it, looking down at all of its filth."

(Pause 5 seconds.)

"And now, I want you to kneel down in front of the disgusting spittoon."

(Pause 5 seconds.)

"As you closely kneel, notice all the filthy, raunchy cigarette butts floating in the disgusting, stinking pool of spit."

(Pause 5 seconds.)

"Now, all that you disgustingly see and smell, right in front of your face, you will *strongly associate* with cigarette smoking. *Do it! Do this association! Now!*"

(Pause 5 seconds.)

"So that, whenever in the future you're just about to light up a cigarette, you'll also strongly experience all the disgust you now feel, from seeing and smelling all the disgusting spit and butts, in this spittoon."

(Pause 5 seconds.)

"And now, push your face into the awful spit and butts, as you *fully experience the awfulness of smoking!*"

(Pause 5 seconds.)

"Feel some of the spit and butts get in your nose and mouth, as you strongly associate all this with cigarette smoking!"

(Pause 5 seconds.)

"Okay, enough! *The experience is over*! You're here in the present, again. The cowboy saloon of 1880 is back in the past, and you're here again, in the present. Your face is *no longer* in the spittoon, and your face, nose, and mouth no longer have any spit or butts in, or on, them; they're *clean*!"

(Pause 5 seconds.)

"But your memory of this disgust will remain strong! You will *strongly associate smoking* with all the disgust of the memory of your face in the spittoon."

(Pause 5 seconds.)

"So that, every time you want a cigarette, the disgusting memory of your face in the spittoon will be *so strong* that it will *completely stop you from smoking!*"

(Pause 5 seconds.)

"Because you will *strongly* associate smoking with the disgusting memory of your face in the spittoon, you'll never smoke again!"

(Pause 5 seconds.)

"In fact, right now, you feel such tremendous disgust towards cigarettes, that *right now, you absolutely know that you will never smoke again*! Feel, right now, this *ultra-*

disgust of cigarettes, so strong in you, that you know you will never smoke again! Feel it! *Strongly! Now!*"

(Pause 5 seconds.)

"After I bring you out of this hypnotic trance, you will *clearly remember* all the *extreme negatives* of cigarette smoking that flowed straight into your mind and emotions without any resistance. You will especially remember that cigarettes are so especially toxic and poisonous, that you *must* stop smoking!"

(Pause 5 seconds.)

"Also, whenever any time in the future, you're about to take *any action* toward resuming smoking, you'll strongly experience the disgusting memory of your face in the sickening spittoon, of spit and butts. This returning memory will be so ultra-disgusting, that no smoking will happen, and *you'll never, ever, smoke again*! I repeat, you will *never, ever, smoke again*!"

(Pause 5 seconds.)

"I'm now about to wake you up, from this hypnotic trance. And, after I do you'll feel fine, rested, and refreshed. I'm going to count back from 5 to 1. And as I count back, you'll slowly wake up. So, "5", you're starting to wake up. And, "4", you're waking up even more. And, "3", you're halfway awake. And, "2", you're almost awake, feeling fine, rested, and refreshed. And, "1!" (*clapping of hands, loudly, here*). You're *awake*, feeling fine, rested and refreshed!

(THIS IS THE END OF THE HYPNOTIC SPEECH.)

Note #1. About 95% of the time, the hypnotic subject *will* wake up from the hypnosis, after you say: "1!", and clap your hands loudly. But, about 5% of the time, they won't wake up. If they don't wake up, then shake them gently, and say their name loudly, followed by "Wake up!" This should do it. But if they still won't wake up, then just leave them be. They'll just fall into a normal sleep or nap, and eventually wake up later, on their own. There is nothing to worry about if this happens! Alternatively, you could wait ten minutes, then shake them again, calling out their name.

Note #2. Because the hypnotic speech is either in your *own* voice (on a recording device), or read to you in your *friend's* voice, it probably will be *very powerful*. Possibly, even more powerful than a professional hypnotist's voice, because you intuitively *trust* your own voice and your friend's voice! Also, it's even possible to repeatedly hypnotize yourself (with this hypnotic speech) *every day* (if you want to). Obviously, frequent repetition, of this hypnotic speech, makes it stronger. I suppose it might be okay to change or alter some of the wording, but only if you know what you're doing (because you, yourself, are a semi-professional). Be extremely careful here! All of this hypnotic wording is going straight into your subconscious mind!

Method #13½ - Self-Hypnosis To Take You To An "Inner Guide" Or "Wise Part Of Yourself" Instead

It's also possible to use the 172 "relax-relax-relax" words (from Method #13) *only* (repeated twice). After this, record suggestions that you'll go (inwardly) to an "inner guide" (or wise part of yourself), who will then tell you how *you* can best stop smoking! This method (or perhaps a combination of methods) may be the *most effective* for you!

In this revised hypnotic speech, after you've had about *five minutes of silence* (to receive your wise messages inwardly), then record (on this revised hypnotic recording) the "waking up" words of counting from "5" to "1".

You can try this *alternative* self-hypnosis instead!

Method #14 - The Banishing Method

With common "twelve-step programs", you usually call on a Higher Power, to help you to stop. This Banishing Method uses a similar strategy, in calling on the same Higher Power, but in a different, more-direct, and personal way.

There exists a very ancient system of higher knowledge and wisdom called the *Cabala*. Of the Cabala's many teachings and rituals, a very, very powerful "rubric ritual" is called the "Lesser Banishing Ritual of the Pentagram". This rubric ritual is *absolutely ideal* for banishing something bad from your life, like smoking.

Now, in doing rituals, you do *not* need a lot of expensive equipment and paraphernalia in order to make the ritual work! Rituals work because of the *"Power of Intention"* of the worker of the ritual. So, my instructions for doing the rubric ritual (to banish smoking from your life) will only involve *inexpensive* props. If you want to add more elaborate or expensive props, you can try:

1. a special, meaningful robe,

2. some kind of altar,

3. a candle,

4. a more-elaborate or expensive wand,

5. a symbolized pentagram or special rug,

6. an elaborate head piece,

7. meaningful jewelry,

8. ritual dance (for example, a special "Stop Smoking Dance" you create),

9. posters or symbols on the walls (perhaps something you create),

10. a room specially set aside only for rituals,

11. appropriate music (perhaps your own recorded "Stop Smoking Song" or "Stop Smoking Chant" that you've created),

12. aroma-therapies or flower essences that increase your "Power of Intention",

13. crystals,

14. Tibetan singing bowls,

15. drumming, flute playing, or playing any instrument you choose,

16. lunar timing (starting at the new moon, etc.),

17. ritual nudity,

18. an ashtray stuffed with smoked butts (symbolizing quitting?) resting on a crushed cigarette pack, perhaps,

19. anything else you can think of, to increase the power of this "Banishing-Smoking Ritual".

Incidentally, rituals are *"advanced working psychology"*, and are somewhat similar to self-hypnosis. In rituals, you are sort of "putting a spell" on yourself or your subconscious mind (in this case, to stop smoking). "Part A" (the part of you that wants to quit) is "putting a ritualistic spell" on "Part B" (the part of you that *won't* quit)! Every day we go through this dichotomy naturally, where different parts of our personality struggle to get their way (over other, opposite, parts of our personality). So, this is all just basic-basic psychology, really. Doing a ritual is just taking it one step further. It's simply more *powerful* to use self-hypnosis, affirmations, chanting, meditating, aromatherapies, yoga, tai-chi, trance-dance, counseling, religion, 12-step programs, or *rituals*, to stop an out-of-control part of our personality from *wrecking our life by smoking*!

For this ritual, you could just use your extended fore-finger, instead of a wand or ritual dagger. Or, you could easily create a special "stop smoking wand" by scotch-taping a crushed, empty cigarette pack to the end of a wooden ruler (or wooden paint-mixing stick). Over this crushed cigarette pack, scotch-tape a huge, cardboard "X" (colored black) that's twice as long, and wide, as the cigarette pack. This "stop smoking wand" graphically symbolizes your intention to quit!

Instructions for Rubric Ritual

1. Face *East*, in the middle of a room, or in front of your altar (optional).

2. Have your wand nearby for later, and ready to pick it up quickly.

3. Touch your forehead, and say (aloud): *"ATAH!"* (Hebrew for "Thou Art".)

4. Touch your solar plexus, and say (aloud): *"MALKUTH!"* (Hebrew for "The Kingdom".)

5. Touch your *right* shoulder and say (aloud): *"VE-GEVURAH!"* (Hebrew for "And the Power".)

6. Touch your *left* shoulder and say (aloud): *"VE-GEDULAH!"* (Hebrew for "And the Glory".)

7. Join your palms together in the common "praying" gesture (fingers pointing up). Put your joined palms over the exact middle of your chest (heart chakra), and say (aloud): *"LE-OLAHM, AMEN!"* (Hebrew for "Forever, Amen".)

8. Pick up your wand (from nearby) and hold it in your dominant hand.

9. Draw a huge five-armed star (a *pentagram*) in the air, with your wand. Imagine the star flaming blue fire, as you draw it. Start at the lower left (1), then move your wand diagonally upward (about four feet) to the star's top-most point (2). Then, move your wand diagonally down to the star's lower right point (3). Then move your wand to the star's left-side point (4). Then, to the star's right-side point (5). Finally, move your wand back diagonally down to the starting point, at the lower left (1). The star is now drawn! All the while, as you draw it, imagine it flaming, in blue fire, in the air!

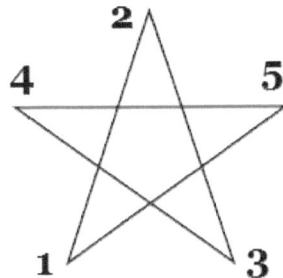

10. Stab the star in its middle with your wand, and say (assertively): *"YOD-HEH-VAV-HEH!"* (This, incidentally, is one of the most powerfully manifesting ritualistic words that exists, as this is the highest Hebrew expression for God's name.)

11. Turn clockwise (to your right), and face *South*. Draw a second star (of flaming blue fire) in the air, as before, stab it in the center, and say (assertively): *"AH-DOH-NAI!"* (Another Hebrew expression, meaning "My Lord", used only for God.)

12. Turn clockwise and face *West*. Draw a third star (of flaming blue fire) in the air, as before, stab it in the center, and say (assertively): *"EH-YEH!"* (Yet another Hebrew name for God.)

13. Turn clockwise, and face *North*. Draw a fourth star (of flaming blue fire) in the air, as before, stab it in the center, and say (assertively): *"AH-GAH-LAH!"* (A Hebrew acronym for *"ATAH GIBOR LE-OLAHM ADONAI"*, meaning "You, O Lord, are mighty forever", used as a name of God.)

14. Turn clockwise (to complete the circle) and Face *East* again (as you started).

15. Hold your arms straight out to the sides, with your wand still in your hand (so that your body forms a cross), and say:

    "*BEFORE ME IS RAPHAEL*

    "*BEHIND ME IS GABRIEL*

    "*TO MY RIGHT IS MICHAEL*

    "*AND TO MY LEFT IS ARIEL*

    "*ABOUT ME FLAME THE PENTAGRAMS*

    "*AND ABOVE ME SHINES THE POWER AND GLORY OF GOD!*"

16. Then say:

    "*ARCHANGEL RAPHAEL! ARCHANGEL GABRIEL!*

    "*ARCHANGEL MICHAEL! ARCHANGEL ARIEL!*

    "*GOD, WITH ALL YOUR POWER AND GLORY!*

    "*PLEASE, HELP ME TO STOP SMOKING, AS QUICKLY AS POSSIBLE!*

    "*PLEASE, I AM ASKING FOR YOUR HELP!*"

17. Intensely *feel* as much *desire* as you possibly can, that you will stop smoking!

18. Then, intensely *feel* as much *triumph* as you possibly can, as you feel strongly confident that you actually will stop!

19. And then, stand there, for about a minute, and *feel* the incredible *spiritual power* of the four highest archangels, and God, empowering you to stop smoking. (If your arms get tired, you can bend them a little, to ease the strain of holding them straight out. You can cup your palms a bit, to receive the Highest Energy from the four archangels and God.)

20. Put down your wand, at the nearby spot where you had it at the start.

21. Touch your forehead, and say (aloud): "*ATAH!*"

22. Touch your solar plexus, and say (aloud): "*MALKUTH!*"

23. Touch your *right* shoulder and say (aloud): "*VE-GEVURAH!*"

24. Touch your *left* shoulder and say (aloud): "*VE-GEDULAH!*"

25. Join your palms together in the common "praying" gesture (fingers pointing up). Put your joined palms over the exact middle of your chest (heart chakra), and say (aloud): "*LE-OLAHM, AMEN!*" (This completes the rubric ritual.)

Aftermath. Feel the powerful effects of this rubric ritual awhile, either as you just stand there, or go and sit down, or lie down. You may feel very spiritual, from your contact with the four archangels and God. You may feel other feelings, or sensations, and it would be good to write all this down in a special notebook, or "Ritual Diary". Also, write down any insights that may come to you, that may creatively help you to stop smoking. These insights and intuitions *could* be very important spiritual messages coming from the four archangels and God, to facilitate your stopping smoking! Be sure to write them down!

Note. If you live in a thin-walled place, where neighbors can easily hear you, it's okay to whisper or softly mumble all the ritual's words. The powerfulness of your *intention* is what's important, not necessarily the loudness of your words!

Doing this rubric ritual daily should greatly help you to quit smoking! You are asking the *Highest Spiritual Forces In The Universe* to help you to quit smoking! Thus, this method is similar to a twelve-step program. The difference is that you can contact God and the four archangels yourself, directly, whenever you want, so that you're creating a personal, intimate relationship with God and the four archangels, as they help you to stop smoking.

Because this "little" rubric ritual seems so "simple" and "brief", many, many people have *completely underestimated its power*! Actually, it's one of the most powerful working rituals ever devised by mankind! For, what could be more powerful than contacting God and the four chief archangels, using all the super-powerful words that are spoken in this rubric ritual?

This Banishing Method can be combined with any other methods to stop smoking. But, *especially* combine it with any intuitions, insights, ideas, or guidance received from God at the conclusion of the rubric ritual. (Write all this down, in your "Ritual Diary".)

Go ahead and *try* this rubric ritual, and you'll be *amazed* to find out how incredibly well it *works*!

[**Caution**. If this ritual doesn't seem to be working after 10 tries, then discontinue it! Afterward, if "God" or any "Archangels" seem to start talking *back* to you, ignore them or tell them to stop. This is because most likely they're autonomous psychological entities you may have created with this ritual. Obviously, *you* need to decide how to live your life, not voices from the subconscious calling themselves "God" or by a name of one the Archangels. Also, anyone with a history of mental illness may need to avoid this method.]

Method #15 - The Anger Method

(By Bill, who smoked for 20 years.)

Bill stopped smoking (finally) with anger! He got *really angry* about all the negatives of cigarettes. Angry about the expense of cigarettes. Angry about being a nicotine addict. Angry about the smoke stinking up his clothes. Angry about it wrecking his health. Angry about smoking in public getting harder and harder, because smoking was banned so often, everywhere. Angry that smoking could eventually kill him. Angry about his constantly craving a cigarette so much. But especially, angry towards all the people who wanted him to quit!

Bill took his *utter volcano of anger*, and turned it towards cigarettes themselves! Bill was so angry about all the negatives of cigarettes, and so *absolutely fed up*, with all the negatives of smoking, that he turned his furious, raging anger towards cigarettes themselves, and was thus able to quit!

For, when furious, boiling anger, that fills your whole being, becomes so incredibly big that you want to kill or destroy something, then it's a very, very powerful thing. And, if you can then turn that powerful, voluminous anger towards something *bad*, then you can destroy that bad thing! And, that's what Bill did. He took his ultra-enormous anger, and directed it towards cigarettes and smoking themselves, and thus was able to quit!

Gary Pickler

Chapter 7 - 45 MINI-METHODS

The Mini-Methods are listed in alphabetical order.

Acupuncture & Acupressure (Mini-Method #1)

Inserting the very fine Chinese needles, in your ears (and upper back?) for twenty minutes, can *really help* with a stop-smoking program! Acupuncture reduces cravings and other withdrawal symptoms. It detoxifies, balances, and relaxes the body. Acupuncture treatments can be a bit expensive without health care coverage for this, but the money you'll save from stopping smoking offsets this! When cravings hit between sessions, pressing tiny balls (taped to acupuncture points) stops these cravings! Also, acu-*pressure* massage can be done on the ears too, by pressing thoroughly, all over each ear, *hitting every single ear acupuncture point* by this method! Try this (thorough) pressing-all-points-on-ears technique. It almost always creates an instant happy mood! This acu-*pressure* can *effectively work*, to stop cigarette cravings, too. Try it, when cravings strike!

Calamus (Acorus calamus, or Sweet Flag Root) (Mini-Method #2)

Calamus calms and centers you. It also stimulates and gives extra energy and stamina. It helps digestion and soothes upset stomach. Calamus can increase appetite, and it helps to clear out lung toxins from smoking. *Chewing calamus root can kill the taste for tobacco*! Try this, to see if this "chewing calamus root" will stop cigarette cravings for you!

Catnip (Mini-Method #3)

Catnip isn't just for cats! Catnip helps calm you, reducing anxiety and insomnia, when you're in the cigarette-quitting stage. Catnip also helps with headache and upset stomach. *Several drops of catnip tincture, on the back of the tongue, can decrease cigarette desire and craving*! Be careful of *excessive* catnip, which can cause nausea, vomiting, or headaches.

Cayenne Pepper (Mini-Method #4)

Cayenne pepper greatly helps you to stop smoking! It produces endorphins that help raise mood, similar to the "mood-raising" of cigarettes. Cayenne helps overcome, and bring down, nicotine cravings. Your lungs become less-sensitive to tobacco's chemical irritants, with cayenne. Cayenne for breakfast reduces appetite (off-setting the tendency to eat more and gain weight when quitting smoking.) Cayenne stimulates the cigarette detox process, by facilitating the excretion of cigarette toxins faster. You can add a few pinches of cayenne to your glass of water. Or, slowly drink warm water with ¼ teaspoon of cayenne, which is very healthful for the heart.

Don't use cayenne if you have stomach ulcers or acidity. Experiment with a little cayenne, in your drink or food. You'll be glad you did!

Citrus Fruits (Mini-Method #5)

Drinking orange or grapefruit juice (or lemonade) can reduce cravings for cigarettes! This is because citrus fruits give you an energetic "kick" that's similar to the smoking "kick". Also, smoking after citrus fruit isn't as pleasant, some people find. In addition, the Vitamin C abundant in fresh (only) citrus fruits can *replenish* Vitamin C that smoking causes to be depleted.

Coltsfoot (Mini-Method #6)

Coltsfoot helps cleanse the lungs by promoting coughing, which expels mucus. Start using at a low dose, to cough only once in awhile. Doses too high, at first, can produce over-coughing, so don't use it if you get so you cannot stop coughing!

Diet (Mini-Method #7)

Eat sensibly, with foods and drinks that nourish your body! Avoid junk foods that just make your withdrawal symptoms worse. Also, avoid sweets, which at first give you a quick "sugar rush", but then lead to severe drops in blood sugar levels, later. A lower blood sugar level, when combined with withdrawal symptoms, will make it *much* harder not to reach for another cigarette!

Try not to eat more, after quitting smoking. Fill up with more fruits and vegetables. Try having small meals, but more frequently. Eat more protein, healthy fats (coconut oil, organic butter, fish) and non-starchy vegetables to give you more energy, that lasts! Eat a well-balanced diet, to give your body the 100 nutrients it needs every day. Eating eggs, yogurt, cheese, fish, and beans, in your meals and snacks, provides essential amino acids, probiotics, and healthy fats that will provide the energy and healthiness you need, to offset any withdrawal symptoms. *Organic foods* in your diet usually give you much more nutrition and fewer toxins, than non-organic foods, and are especially needed by your body at this time. Focus on eating the very healthiest, now!

Dream Solution Method (Mini-Method #8)

Before going to bed at night, write down these words, and put them under your pillow: "I wish for my dream tonight to inspire me with the *best solution*, for me to stop smoking!" (Word this message in your own way, if you want.)

After you put your "dream solution message" under your pillow, feel *extreme desire* for this to happen. You can light a candle, look at the candle, and *feel burning desire* that you'll receive (in your dream) guidance, of what's the best way for you to stop smoking!

Then, feel *extreme triumph*, the "winning feeling", as if *you have already received* (from the dream) the guidance of how to best stop smoking! Then, put out the candle, and retire for the night.

If you wake up in the middle of the night (or in the morning) with your dream's "stop smoking solution", be sure to write it down! (Have pen and paper, and a light, easily reachable from your bed.) Or, if after a week of trying this every night, you still haven't received a "guidance dream", then try taking some *herbs* that stimulate dreaming, before going to sleep. Do an Internet search on "dreaming herbs that stimulate dreaming", to find herbs that seem to be best for this, or try the "Dream Enhancer" formula of 1/8 teaspoon each of the dried herbs: valerian, hops, and skullcap. Or, you can buy a Native American "dream catcher" talisman, which also could help; search online for this, too!

Vision Quest & Lucid Dreaming (Mini-Method #8½)

Going on a Native American "Vision Quest" could give you the solution (of how to best stop smoking). Do a "Vision Quest" computer search, to learn how. Or, you could experiment with "Lucid Dreaming", where you do techniques to "wake up" in a dream, yet stay in the dream world (with your awake mind). Then, search in the "lucid dream world" for a guru, wise person, or shaman, who will tell you how to best stop smoking. Ophiel's book *The Art and Practice of Astral Projection*, has a "dream method" that leads to "awakening in your dream".

H.P. Lovecraft once wrote an *incredible* short story entitled *The Dream Quest of the Unknown Kadath*. The hero of this story, in a lucid dream state, searches for (and finds) the "realm of the gods", where he finally receives the answers that he seeks! Reading this amazing story may inspire you to try a similar quest yourself, for your "stop smoking" solutions.

Anyway, this "Lucid Dreaming" method is definitely worth a try, since your own *personal* answer, of how to best stop smoking, may simply *lie within* you!

Echinacea (Mini-Method #9)

Echinacea helps stop infection, disease, fever, and blood poisoning that might result from cigarette toxins overwhelming your body, as they're eliminated from your body, when you quit smoking.

Elderberry Flower (Mini-Method #10)

It helps reduce any inflammation of the lungs, or bronchial tubes, that can occur from stopping smoking.

Eleuthero Root (Mini-Method #11)

This herb helps to turn around any stress and fatigue resulting from quitting smoking. Also, it strengthens the immune system.

Flower Essences (Mini-Method #12)

A soothing, calming effect is brought about by Bach Rescue Remedy. It's very stress-reducing and relaxing. It really helps in turning around the extreme stress of cigarette withdrawal. There are many other flower essences that can help here, too. Experiment with several promising-looking ones, to find the best ones that work for *you*, in your stressful cigarette withdrawal.

Ginger Root (Mini-Method #13)

Ginger root helps to stop and relieve any nausea, which sometimes results from cigarette withdrawal.

Ginseng (Mini-Method #14)

Nibbling on a ginseng root can be something else to put in your mouth, besides a cigarette. Chewing one or two grams, off the end of a root, delivers a standard daily dose. Ginseng can be subtle, but it tonifies, energizes, and increases alertness. A standardized extract of 4% to 7% ginsenosides seems to give the best results and benefits.

Ginseng helps you deal much better with the stress of stopping smoking. Physical endurance and stamina are increased during your smoking withdrawal period. Ginseng reduces anxiety and improves mood. Ginseng helps rebuild the lungs, and reduces worry.

With ginseng powder, try adding a teaspoon to your morning meal, to help cut down cigarette cravings!

Ginseng needs to be taken for two weeks, then *not taken* for two weeks! Taking ginseng with *ginger* helps a lot, too. With this schedule of "two weeks on, and two weeks off" ginseng, you avoid any possible "ginseng overdose" side effects.

Take ginseng before noon, or its energizing properties may interfere with your *sleep* that night (if taken after noon).

Ginseng, for several reasons, can be an excellent help, in any stop smoking program!

Grape Juice (Mini-Method #15)

When you drink it daily, grape juice greatly helps to flush out nicotine and other cigarette chemicals from the body. Use it after quitting smoking.

Grape Seed Extract (Mini-Method #16)

It helps to heal any lung damage caused by cigarette smoking.

Herbal Cigarettes (Mini-Method #17)

Herbal cigarettes usually have herbs like licorice, cinnamon, mint, cornsilk, cloves, lemongrass, tea leaves, ginseng, and various other non-tobacco products. Herbal cigarettes can help break tobacco addiction, because they satisfy your psychological need to smoke, without being addictive or being anywhere near as bad for you, as tobacco! Often they're just a short-term, healthy replacement, to stopping the tobacco habit. Herbal cigarettes help your lungs expel the toxic build-up, from tobacco smoking.

Herbalist Howie Brounstein recommends this 7-herb mixture, to help quit smoking: rubbed mullein leaf, kinnikinnik (bearberry) leaf, manzanita leaf, skullcap leaf, lobelia leaf, coltsfoot leaf (and peppermint leaf and/or spearmint leaf only if you smoked menthols).

Break up the kinnikinnik and manzanita into five pieces. After a couple of weeks, reduce or stop the lobelia.

For more information, read *The Preparation of Herbs into a Palatable Smoking Mixture*. Skullcap, turmeric, passion-flower, and elderberry can also be added to a smoking mixture.

Herbal cigarettes can be bought online, or even (perhaps) at your local tobacco shop. Here are four types of herbal cigarettes that can be ordered, at one site:

1) Clove Herbal Cigarettes (heavy type feel, with a bit of a sweet taste).

2) Menthol Cigarettes (specially blended herbs, with cool menthol taste).

3) Honey Rose (herbs include marshmallow, red clover, and rose, with honey).

4) Ginseng Herbal Cigarettes.

One pack is $5.50. One carton is $50.00.

Go to the website *Herbal Cigarettes - Quit Smoking / Just Another WordPress Site*, to order,

or http://HerbalCigarettesOnline.com.

When smoking herbal cigarettes, do not "cheat" and slip in a tobacco cigarette now and then, or you'll just continue to be addicted to tobacco. But if this urge to "cheat" becomes too strong, add some lobelia to your herbal smoking mixture, so that lobelia's main active ingredient, lobeline, will stimulate your brain much like nicotine, but it's a lot less harmful.

Go ahead and experiment with different blends of herbal cigarettes, until you find a mixture that will work, for you!

Homeopathy (Mini-Method #18)

Pre-made formulas on the market, like "Smoker's Calm" and "Stop-it Smoking", help. Some people are very affected by homeopathy remedies, while others feel no effects at all. But, they're worth a try, since they have no side effects.

Honey (Mini-Method #19)

Honey helps to ease cigarette withdrawal, with all of its health-giving vitamins and enzymes.

Horehound (Mini-Method #20)

Horehound helps flush out tar, and other cigarette chemicals, from the lungs and body.

Hypnotherapy (Mini-Method #21)

This author's experience, in hypnotizing many people to stop smoking, was that only 25% of people, who could go into a *deep* trance, actually stopped. The other 75%, who could only go into a *shallow* trance, didn't stop. However, none of my former hypnotic sessions included the extremely powerful "spittoon" technique, of Method #13, the "Hypnotic Ultra-Disgust Method". Probably the success rate will increase to much more than 25%, if the "spittoon" technique is used!

Also, if you use your own voice, or that of a trusted friend, it is more likely that you can relax into a *deep* trance.

If you go to a professional hypnotherapist, try to find one who's either inexpensive (in case it doesn't work), or one who will refund your money, if his/her hypnotherapy fails to stop your smoking. Or, consider making your own self-hypnotic tape, to try.

Hyssop (Mini-Method #22)

Hyssop (an herb) helps in stopping smoking, in the following ways:

1) It alleviates any anxiety or hysteria, which sometimes come with smoking withdrawal.

2) It helps with any stress, from quitting smoking.

3) It relaxes the nervous system.

4) It helps lessen withdrawal symptoms.

5) It clears the lungs and soothes irritated lung membranes.

6) It clears toxins from the lungs, and the rest of the body, brought in by smoking.

Hyssop *can* be a laxative, for some, and cause loose bowels, so try taking a milder dose if this happens.

Licorice Sticks (Mini-Method #23)

The oral habit of smoking can be offset and satisfied by chewing on sticks of licorice root (not the candy). Try chewing on these instead, when you crave a cigarette. Having one in your mouth is a good substitute for a cigarette. Licorice sticks can be bought at herbal shops, or health food stores.

After using licorice for 4 to 6 weeks, discontinue for 2 weeks, before starting up again. This allows your body to recover and re-balance from licorice long-term use.

Licorice also soothes irritation in the lungs, caused by smoking.

Lobelia (Mini-Method #24)

Lobelia is also known as Indian Tobacco. It can be smoked either alone, or mixed-in with other herbs. Lobelia is a very effective herb to stop smoking, because its main active ingredient (lobeline) has an effect, similar to nicotine, on the brain! In fact, lobelia *almost guarantees* success in stopping smoking, due to its lobeline satisfying your *nicotine* cravings, in an alternative way! Also, lobelia's *lobeline* increases the brain's dopamine levels, just like cigarettes do. Lobelia isn't habit-forming or addictive, and lobelia doesn't cause the damage that nicotine does. Also in lobelia is *isolobeline*, which relaxes, eases tension, and calms the nerves. Lobelia helps clear the lungs, too.

Taking 5 to 10 drops of *lobelia tincture* under the tongue, or sipping *lobelia tea*, can stop bad cigarette cravings, within 5 minutes! The taste of lobelia is rather unpleasant, which is why lobelia is often mixed with better-tasting herbs, or perhaps honey (lobelia tea with *lots* of honey in it).

Don't take too much lobelia, or larger amounts may be *slightly* toxic to you (however, compared to tobacco, there isn't too much to worry about, here). You'll be alerted that your amount of lobelia is too high, if you experience: nausea, vomiting, dry mouth, lightheadedness, dizziness, loose bowels, or confusion.

The *best "lobelia strategy"* is to start with a smaller dose, and increase the dose until any side effect (like nausea) is felt. Then, decrease the dose the next day, until the amount of lobelia you take no longer causes any nausea, or other side effect.

Most "authorities on herbs" discourage the taking of lobelia if you have high blood pressure, or heart disease. But, if not taking lobelia means smoking tobacco *instead*, then it probably would be slightly better, on your blood pressure and heart, to be smoking lobelia instead of tobacco! (Especially, if you plan to gradually diminish the amount of lobelia, over time.)

Lobelia is *probably the very best solution* (to stop smoking), of all 46 of the Mini-Methods, listed here in this book!

Lobelia *Herb* Combined With "Nicotinic Acid" / Vitamin B-3 (Mini-Method #24-A)

Remember how, earlier in this book (in the chapters describing the Silica System), I informed you that Vitamin B-3, when it was first discovered, was called "Nicotinic Acid"? This was because, when "Nicotinic Acid" enters the body and becomes oxidized, then it has *exactly the same effect, on a person, as nicotine*! (Anthony Shkreli explains this in his books, in much greater detail, for those who want to investigate this more deeply.) Anyway, the original name of Vitamin B-3, "Nicotinic Acid", was later changed to *niacin,* or the related molecule, *niacinamide.*

Well, since lobelia's main active ingredient, *lobeline,* has a similar effect to nicotine, on the brain, why not *combine* lobelia with Vitamin B-3? *"Nicotinic Acid"* (which has a nicotine-like effect, once it enters the body and becomes oxidized)? Of course, as explained earlier in this book, all the B-Vitamins work together, so you'll need to take a Multi-B Vitamin, *with all eleven* (11) B-Vitamins in it[4]. Thus, this "combination method" means, *taking lobelia with a Multi-B Vitamin.* Try it!

Lobelia *Tincture* Combined With "Nicotinic Acid" (Vitamin B-3) (Mini-Method #24-B)

This might be the *ideal combination,* in quickly reducing cigarette cravings! Along with 5 to 10 drops of *lobelia tincture* under the tongue (or sipping *lobelia tea*), take a Vitamin B-3 dose (capsule or pill) of *niacinamide* (*not niacin*), along with

---

4 Preferably with Vitamin B3 in the form of niacinamide instead of niacin, to avoid niacin's very unpleasant flush effect.

a Multi-B Vitamin (with all eleven B-Vitamins in it). The reason you're taking niacinamide and *not* niacin, is that niacin will cause a strong, unpleasant red flush in your face and/or all over your body (perhaps combined with a strong, itching sensation), for perhaps 20 minutes until it fades out. *Avoid* this *very unpleasant* feeling and take Vitamin B-3 as niacinamide, *not* as niacin!

For perhaps three days, you can take a Vitamin B-3 pill of *niacinamide*, in addition to the Multi-B Vitamin! But after three days, you'll probably need to take *only* the Multi-B Vitamin! This is because, for three days, you've been taking *much more Vitamin B-3* (as niacinamide) than all the other B-Vitamins. So, that, after these three days, you're *beginning* to get *deficient*, or have an imbalance, in all the other B-Vitamins, from taking *extra* Vitamin B-3 (niacinamide)! But, if you discontinue the separate Vitamin B-3 dose after three days, you'll stop the imbalance and be fine.

Anyway, in three days, you can *seriously reduce greatly your cigarette cravings*, with the combination of *lobelia tincture* (or *lobelia tea*) plus a Vitamin B-3 (niacinamide) capsule or pill, plus a Multi-B Vitamin capsule or pill. (Always keep all B-Vitamins in the refrigerator, to keep them fresh!) Then, starting on the fourth day, stop taking the Vitamin B-3 (niacinamide) capsule or pill and combine the lobelia tincture (or lobelia tea) with just the Multi-B Vitamin capsule or pill *only*. This should really "do the trick" of *greatly stopping your nicotine cravings—fast!*

Milk Thistle (Mini-Method #25)

Milk thistle helps the liver in many ways, when stopping smoking, by preventing toxic chemicals from entering liver cells. Daily, take 420 mg (milligrams) of "silymarin" (standardized milk thistle extract), dividing into three doses, using a "standardized" milk thistle product.

Mimosa (Mini-Method #26)

This herb helps reduce anxiety and headaches, which can result from stopping cigarettes.

Mindfulness Meditation (Mini-Method #27)

This helps soothe away the stress of withdrawal symptoms. Sit in a comfortable, quiet place, without distraction. Perhaps wear earplugs, to block out stressful noise. Perhaps wear green, color-therapy glasses, which are very restful and relaxing. Repeat a soothing "mantra" over and over (the mantra "I-YING, I-YING, I-YING", etc., works well), or "watch" (pay attention to) your breath (as in Vipassana meditation). Experiment with different meditations, to find out what works best, for you. Scientific books on mindfulness meditation have been written by Jon Kabat-Zinn, Ph.D., and Herbert Benson, M.D., if you would like to learn more why this method can be very helpful!

Rajneesh, or Osho, wrote about numerous good meditation techniques. Searching on the Internet can uncover at least a *dozen* different types of meditation, to experiment with.

Mullein (Mini-Method #28)

This herb helps to soothe irritation and inflammation in the lungs, when quitting cigarettes. It helps heal the lungs' mucus membranes. Mullein also is a gentle sedative that calms you, reducing anxiety and insomnia. Mullein can be added to other herbs to smoke, in weaning yourself off cigarettes.

Nicotine Replacement Therapy (Mini-Method #29)

Nicotine patches and gums can be effective, for some people. Also, the *Electronic Cigarette (Mini-Method #29½)* can be helpful. You can switch to these, then gradually wean yourself off them, with the aid of other methods mentioned in this book. Better success often occurs with a combination of different methods!

Nutritional Supplements (Mini-Method #30)

Taking Vitamins A, C, and E replenishes any deficiency of them caused by smoking—a likely deficiency, since *each cigarette uses up a full-day's requirement of Vitamin C!*

Also, Vitamins A, C, D, and E help in coping with cigarette withdrawal symptoms. A B-Vitamin capsule, pill, or powder (always keep B-Vitamins in your refrigerator!) that contains all eleven B-Vitamins, will help greatly.

A Multi-Mineral supplement (capsule, powder, or liquid) is good, too, and should include at least as much magnesium as calcium in it. Some people need twice as much magnesium as calcium, especially if you have "B" Blood Type. Some people need twice as much calcium as magnesium, but calcium is easier to get from food. A good Multi-Mineral supplement will also have chromium, selenium, and zinc, as well as trace minerals. Our body needs 100 nutrients daily, and about 60 of these are minerals! Natural Sea Salt has all of the minerals.

All of these vitamins and minerals will greatly help your health and energy, and will lessen the impact of withdrawal symptoms!

Oat Extract (Mini-Method #31)

An extract of green oats, called "wild oats" or "oat grass", can help ease withdrawal symptoms from, and reduce cravings for, cigarettes. Oat extracts reduce stress and anxiety, tonify the nervous system, and help reduce insomnia.

Oats themselves are rich in the amino acid L-Tryptophan, which helps the body produce serotonin, a "feel-good" body chemical, which helps alleviate depression and create a happier mood. However, chicken has much more L-Tryptophan, should you need to supplement your diet with this necessary nutrient (organic *only* chicken would be recommended).

Wild oat extract, or tea, has high medicinal value and is completely safe, even when doing it long-term. Since oats themselves have gluten, they are not recommended in large amounts, or on a daily basis.

Passion Flower (Mini-Method #32)

This herb helps to calm, relax, and help relieve insomnia. It helps to reduce irritability and restlessness from cigarette withdrawal. It reduces nicotine cravings. Passion Flower can be included, with other herbs, in an herbal smoking mixture, used for weaning from cigarettes. (See *Mini-Method #17*.)

Peppermint Leaf (Mini-Method #33)

It helps to detox you, when quitting smoking. It also helps you relax more.

Plantain (Mini-Method #34)

This herb makes you not want to smoke cigarettes. Plantain can either be ingested, or sprayed up your nostrils. Plantain soothes mucus membranes (including lungs) that have been irritated by smoking.

Radish (Mini-Method #35)

Grate a radish, and mix the juice with honey. Drink it at least twice a day, to provide another "home remedy" for stopping smoking.

Rhodiola (Mini-Method #36)

This herb reduces withdrawal symptoms from quitting smoking. It helps you to cope with physical, environmental, and mental stress. It helps burn fat, from any weight gain, from quitting smoking. It strengthens the mind, and improves mood. Doses range from 200 mg to 600 mg. Adjust your dose according to your symptoms.

Safflower Herb (Mini-Method #37)

Safflower herb helps the whole "stop smoking process", due to its anti-tumor properties.

Set A Quit-Date (Mini-Method #38)

Set a quit-date, and tell others who support you. This helps you to prepare for quitting, in all ways! Choose a day when you're not at work. Vince Stead (see Method #2) quit on his father's birthday, perhaps activating the Freudian Superego (internalized parental figure) to ally with him, in his efforts to quit.

Skullcap Herb (Mini-Method #39)

Skullcap helps to calm and heal the brain and nervous system, when you quit smoking. It treats anxiety, nervousness, and insomnia. It reduces tension and stress. But, skullcap can also make you drowsy, so don't use it when alertness is needed. (Skullcap herb is also used in Mini-Method #8.)

St. John's Wort (Mini-Method #40)

These are all the ways that St. John's Wort can help:

1) It soothes cigarette withdrawal symptoms.

2) It helps quench tobacco cravings.

3) It calms and relaxes.

4) It heals lung damage, from smoking.

5) It increases dopamine levels, to offset cigarette cravings. (Dopamine is a body chemical that induces happy moods.)

6) It helps eliminate toxins in your blood that were introduced there by smoking.

7) It restores the balance between serotonin and dopamine in the brain.

8) It has hypericin, which is its most-significant ingredient.

9) It treats anxiety, melancholy, and depression.

10) It helps insomnia and nervousness.

11) It is an effective alternative remedy to Prozac and similar drugs; it costs less and is safer.

12) It is non-addictive, has no side effects, and therefore is preferred over many patented drugs with their synthetic, patented molecules.

Some words of advice, when taking St. John's Wort, are:

1) It can sometimes take 2 to 3 weeks to notice its effects.

2) It makes you more-vulnerable to sunburn, so *do not stay in the sun any longer* than makes your skin a tiny bit pink, and avoid early-morning and late-afternoon sun rays, which are more red.

The best dose of St. John's Wort seems to be 300 mg, taken 3 times daily. Also possible is 450 mg, taken twice a day. St. John's Wort supplements can easily be bought over-the-counter and come as: oil, tincture, or capsule.

Try it! It really works!

Steam-Sweating Shower (Mini-Method #41)

When you quit smoking, all the hundreds of toxins (from the cigarettes) try to leave your body! This is one of the reasons why you feel so *miserable*, as the toxins go to your liver and kidneys, etc. Well, by sweating lots, in a hot shower, you can sweat a lot of the toxins out your skin, preventing them from going through your liver or kidneys!

Instructions for a Steam-Sweating Shower:

1) Cover your head with a towel dipped in cold water, and then squeezed out. It's a sort of "turban" you wear, to protect your brain from the extreme heat.

2) Take as hot a shower as your skin can possibly stand. As you do this, scrub your skin with a wash rag and a soap that absolutely *does not clog your skin's pores*! Don't use any soap with deodorant or additives or chemicals, which all clog your skin's pores, which reduces sweating! Recommended is either a natural soap or Ivory soap. Alternatively, using *Planet* brand *dishwashing liquid* is OK, because it will not clog pores and is certified to biodegrade to water, carbon dioxide, and healthful minerals.

3) Stand in the shower's hot water, after washing off the soap, for about ten minutes, as you sweat and sweat and sweat! (It's possible for you to be sitting on a small stool here, instead of standing.) Have the hot water run down your back, as you stand or sit.

4) After ten minutes, turn the shower's water to *cold* (or as cold as you can stand it).

5) Scrub yourself off a second time, with the wash rag and soap, to remove all the oily sweat accumulated on the

surface of your skin (that will harden, and feel terrible, if not scrubbed off in this second wash-rag scrubbing).

6) Step out of your "steam-sweating" shower, dry off, and feel how *good* your skin feels, and how much better *you* feel (from sweating out all those cigarette toxins and washing them away).

7) Drink plenty of water (filtered water is best), and eat some nourishing raw fruits or vegetables, to rebuild electrolyte and blood-nutrient levels (you may feel a little "tipsy", after all the sweating), and then some healthy protein and fats.

8) Don't drive your car for awhile, until you feel completely back to normal again, from eating healthy foods to rebuild nutrients that may have been sweated-out, along with the toxins.

Note. Do *not* do this steam-sweating shower if you have a *weak heart*! High water-temperatures in a shower, with a long session of sweating, can overly strain a weak heart!

Support Network Creation (Mini-Method #42)

Include friends, and possibly family, to support your quitting. Perhaps even start a "Stop-Smoking Support Network Group", with an ad on a bulletin board, on Craig's List, Facebook, etc. Join up with special other people, who you can telephone, if you feel your resolve weakening. Find others who have quit! Then, try their method, with their support. "Quit-Smoking Programs" can offer you extra support. Some of these are even free of charge. Ask around for them, or find them with an Internet search.

Think Positive, Keep Busy (Mini-Method #43)

Using positive thinking—confirming that you are *actually able to quit*—works much better than negative thinking, here!

Do all your favorite activities, keeping you very busy, to distract from your cigarette cravings. Instead of a cigarette, put either of the following in your mouth: gum, candy, a toothpick, a licorice stick, a ginseng root, a pencil or pen, or celery and carrot sticks (with favorite dip), a straw, etc.

Keep your fingers and hands busy with alternate activities to cigarette lighting and holding. Use your hands to play around with rubber bands, pens, pencils, rings, jewelry, watches, balls, toys (like *kendama* or *yoyo*), brain teasers (like disentanglement puzzles, Rubik's Cube, disentanglement puzzles, 3D mazes, etc.), solitaire (card game), petting pets, stroking your hair, face or arms, etc. Alternatively, *massage* different parts of your body: ears, hand, feet, lower back (reaching around), etc.

Never let the temptation to "smoke just one more" wreck your whole stop-smoking program!

Turmeric In Abundance (Mini-Method #43½)

Eat as much turmeric powder as you comfortably can, with meals. Or take lots and lots of turmeric capsules with meals. Turmeric is incredibly silica-rich. And silica stops all craving to smoke. See section Turmeric-Powder-Power in Chapter 2.

Add 1/10 teaspoon of *organic black pepper* to each level teaspoon of turmeric powder. This will increase the absorption and effectiveness of the turmeric powder *greatly!*

Valerian Root (Mini-Method #44)

How valerian root helps:

1) It reduces stress, irritability, nervous tension, and anxiety, which are often experienced during stopping smoking.

2) It stops insomnia and helps you to get to sleep, from any sleeplessness resulting from stopping smoking.

3) It slightly sedates you. This calming effect offsets the stress and anxiety caused by nicotine cravings.

4) It has been taken for centuries for anti-anxiety, ever since the times of ancient Rome and Greece.

5) It also helps to relax the muscles, soothing stress.

Beware of large doses, which may cause dizziness or drowsiness. Don't drive a car after taking valerian root, and consider using valerian root only in the evenings.

Valerian root is easily available in health food stores or herbal shops, in capsule form. Or, you can make a tea from 2 to 3 grams of valerian root, in hot water. (Valerian root is also used in Mini-Method #8.)

Water (Mini-Method #45)

Water helps to detox the body, when quitting cigarettes. Drink a glass of water (filtered or reverse-osmosis water is best) instead, when you crave a cigarette.

If you have issues with gaining weight as you stop smoking, drink a pint of water before every meal, to cut down on over-eating.

"Way of Random Choice" (Mini-Method #46)

This is for those who can't make up their mind, of which of the 15 methods and 45 other mini-methods to try! All of these methods and mini-methods are just too overwhelming to some people! Well, instead of just throwing your hands in the air, in confusion and indecision, perhaps you could let a series of six coin-flips decide which of the 60 possibilities to try first!

Instructions:

1) Take out a quarter, and sit in front of a large empty table. (This can also be done by flipping a coin onto the floor.)

2) Flip the quarter with your thumb, up into the air above the table, so that it rapidly turns over and over, many times, before landing on the table. (If it falls onto the floor, it still counts, heads or tails.)

3) Record whether it's a "head" or "tail" with an "H" or "T".

4) Do this six times in total, to have a series of "H"-s or "T"-s written down. *For example*, it might be "H T T H T H."

5) *Match up your series of letters to the list below, and you have your first random choice!*

6) If you like this choice of a Method or Mini-Method, then go ahead and start using it, to stop smoking!

7) *If you don't really like* what has randomly come up, then go back to Step (2), and try it all again, with six more coin-flips.

8) Keep doing the six-coin-flip-series, until you get a Method or Mini-Method that you like enough to *actually begin doing, starting today!*

9) You may need to keep going, with your six-coin-flip-series, until you have *three* Methods or Mini-Methods *to do in combination!* This is because a combination of three (Methods or Mini-Methods) can be more powerful and effective.

Six-Coin-Flip-Series, Matched Up With Methods & Mini-Methods:

H–H–H–H–H–H	Method #1: The Silica System
H–H–H–H–H–T	Method #2: Sicken Yourself With Cigs
H–H–H–H–T–H	Method #3: Affirm Quitting Date Repeatedly, As One Smokes Heavily And Excessively
H–H–H–H–T–T	Method #4: Very Gradual Reduction Of 'The Patch"
H–H–H–T–H–H	Method #5: Weaning
H–H–H–T–H–T	Method #6: Top Notch, Competent Counseling
H–H–H–T–T–H	Method #7: Lobelia
H–H–H–T–T–T	Method #8: Herbal Blends
H–H–T–H–H–H	Method #9: Herbal Tea Of Silica-Rich Herbs

H–H–T–H–H–T	Method #10: Stop In 3 Days: Methods #1 Through #9 Combined
H–H–T–H–T–H	Method #11: Limit Of 7-A-Day System
H–H–T–H–T–T	Method #12: The Fear-Of-Death Method
H–H–T–T–H–H	Method #13: Hypnotic Ultra-Disgust Method
H–H–T–T–H–T	Method #13½: Self-Hypnotic Inner Guide Wisdom Method
H–H–T–T–T–H	Method #14: The Banishing Method!
H–H–T–T–T–T	Method #15: The Anger Method
H–T–H–H–H–H	Mini-Method #1: Acupuncture & Acupressure
H–T–H–H–H–T	Mini-Method #2: Calamus
H–T–H–H–T–H	Mini-Method #3: Catnip
H–T–H–H–T–T	Mini-Method #4: Cayenne Pepper
H–T–H–T–H–H	Mini-Method #5: Citrus Fruits
H–T–H–T–H–T	Mini-Method #6: Coltsfoot
H–T–H–T–T–H	Mini-Method #7: Diet
H–T–H–T–T–T	Mini-Method #8: Dream Solution Method
H–T–T–H–H–H	Mini-Method #8½: Vision Quest & Lucid Dreaming
H–T–T–H–H–T	Mini-Method #9: Echinacea
H–T–T–H–T–H	Mini-Method #10: Elderberry Flower
H–T–T–H–T–T	Mini-Method #11: Eleuthero Root
H–T–T–T–H–H	Mini-Method #12: Flower Essences
H–T–T–T–H–T	Mini-Method #13: Ginger Root

H-T-T-T-T-H	Mini-Method #14: Ginseng
H-T-T-T-T-T	Mini-Method #15: Grape Juice
T-H-H-H-H-H	Mini-Method #16: Grape Seed Extract
T-H-H-H-H-T	Mini-Method #17: Herbal Cigarettes
T-H-H-H-T-H	Mini-Method #18: Homeopathy
T-H-H-H-T-T	Mini-Method #19: Honey
T-H-H-T-H-H	Mini-Method #20: Horehound
T-H-H-T-H-T	Mini-Method #21: Hypnotherapy
T-H-H-T-T-H	Mini-Method #22: Hyssop
T-H-H-T-T-T	Mini-Method #23: Licorice Sticks
T-H-T-H-H-H	Mini-Method #24: Lobelia
T-H-T-H-H-T	Mini-Method #24½ (A or B): Lobelia/ Tincture Combined With Vitamin B-3
T-H-T-H-T-H	Mini-Method #25: Milk Thistle
T-H-T-H-T-T	Mini-Method #26: Mimosa
T-H-T-T-H-H	Mini-Method #27: Mindfulness Meditation
T-H-T-T-H-T	Mini-Method #28: Mullein
T-H-T-T-T-H	Mini-Method #29: Nicotine Replacement: Patches/Gums
T-H-T-T-T-T	Mini-Method #29½: Nicotine Replacement: Electronic Cigarettes
T-T-H-H-H-H	Mini-Method #30: Nutritional Supplements
T-T-H-H-H-T	Mini-Method #31: Oat Extract
T-T-H-H-T-H	Mini-Method #32: Passionflower

T–T–H–H–T–T	Mini-Method #33: Peppermint Leaf
T–T–H–T–H–H	Mini-Method #34: Plantain
T–T–H–T–H–T	Mini-Method #35: Radish
T–T–H–T–T–H	Mini-Method #36: Rhodiola
T–T–H–T–T–T	Mini-Method #37: Safflower Herb
T–T–T–H–H–H	Mini-Method #38: Set A Quit-Date
T–T–T–H–H–T	Mini-Method #39: Skullcap
T–T–T–H–T–H	Mini-Method #40: St. John's Wort
T–T–T–H–T–T	Mini-Method #41: Steam-Sweating Shower
T–T–T–T–H–H	Mini-Method #42: Support Network Creation
T–T–T–T–H–T	Mini-Method #43: Think Positive, Keep Busy
<no code>[5]	Mini-Method #43½: Turmeric-Powder In Abundance Method
T–T–T–T–T–H	Mini-Method #44: Valerian Root
T–T–T–T–T–T	Mini-Method #45: Water

Table 1. Linking H-T combinations with Methods.

Of course, most rational, logical, scientifically minded people would say that one should choose one of the 15 Methods (or 45 Mini-Methods) by:

1. analysis and logic, or

2. emotional appeal, or

3. practicality and common sense.

---

5   If tired of flipping coins, try Mini-Method 43½!

But, who knows? Perhaps choosing by this "Way of Random Choice" might be equally effective! Consider trying it!

Obviously, it's not "either-or" here. Thus, choice of Method (or Mini-Method) can *primarily* be by your usual, personality-based, way of deciding things. Then, a *secondary* choice can be made by this "Way of Random Choice" method. And then perhaps your *primary choice*, and your *secondary choice*, can be combined?

Anyway, your use of this "Way of Random Choice" method is (obviously) completely up to you. Good luck!

CHAPTER 8 - A Smoke-free Future

MORE METHODS NEEDED! PLEASE!

I believe that the best way, to help people to stop smoking, is to provide them with *lots and lots* of methods that actually work! Then, people can choose the method that works for them, *do* this method, and stop!

If you know of *any* other method to stop smoking, *please* let me know of it! Or, if you tried a *combination* of methods in this book that worked, then email *that combination* to me. Send to my email: garypickler1@gmail.com. Thank you!

When I receive fifteen or more methods from you and others, I will write a second book, *15 More Methods To Stop Smoking Fast!*, and all contributors will get a free copy.

Let's get these "stop smoking methods" out into the world, as fast as we can, to help all the smokers who are trapped in their nicotine addiction!

Also, if you liked this book, *please* give it a 5-star review, to encourage others to get it and let it work for them, too! Thank you, thank you, so much!

Conclusion

I've certainly provided you with a wealth of various options and combinations here, haven't I? This is because everyone is different, and thus needs a different "concoction" or formula to successfully carry out the very complicated process of quitting!

So, *choose* your individual method, or personal combination of systems, and leave your smoking habit "in the dust" forever!

However, if at the very, very end of this book, you're still undecided about what to do, and need the *simplest possible solution*, then just eat as much organic turmeric powder (or turmeric powder capsules) as you comfortably can, with all your meals. Turmeric is incredibly silica-rich, and *silica absolutely stops all craving to smoke.*

Be sure to add 1/10 teaspoon of *organic black pepper* to each level teaspoon of turmeric powder. This will increase the absorption and effectiveness of the turmeric powder greatly.

Very effective here is a *tea* of 2 tsp turmeric powder, 1/5 tsp black pepper, 1 tsp olive oil or coconut oil, and 1 tsp honey (or agave nectar, or maple syrup).

This *definitely* will do it; the simplest solution is often the best!

Stop Smoking Fast! 15 Ways That Actually Work.

www.ingramcontent.com/pod-product-compliance
Lightning Source LLC
Chambersburg PA
CBHW021547290526
45785CB00004BA/1949